The Washington Manual® of Bedside Procedures

EDITOR

James Matthew Freer, MD

Assistant Professor
Director, Procedure Service
Division of Hospital Medicine
Department of Internal Medicine
Washington University School of Medicine
St. Louis, Missouri

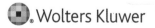 Wolters Kluwer

Philadelphia • Baltimore • New York • London
Buenos Aires • Hong Kong • Sydney • Tokyo

Executive Editor: Rebecca Gaertner
Senior Product Development Editor: Kristina Oberle
Senior Production Project Manager: Cynthia Rudy
Marketing Manager: Stephanie Kindlick
Design Coordinator: Joan Wendt
Senior Manufacturing Coordinator: Beth Welsh
Prepress Vendor: S4Carlisle Publishing Services

9 8 7 6 5 4 3 2 1

Printed in China

Library of Congress Cataloging-in-Publication Data

Names: Freer, James Matthew, editor, contributor. | Washington University (Saint Louis, Mo.). Department of Medicine, issuing body.
Title: The Washington manual of bedside procedures / [edited by] James Matthew Freer.
Other titles: Manual of bedside procedures
Description: First edition. | Philadelphia : Wolters Kluwer Health, [2016] | Includes bibliographical references and index.
Identifiers: LCCN 2015040254 | ISBN 9781496323705 (spiral bound : alk. paper)
Subjects: | MESH: Minor Surgical Procedures—Handbooks. | Diagnostic Techniques, Surgical—Handbooks.
Classification: LCC RD110 | NLM WO 39 | DDC 617/.024—dc23 LC record available at http://lccn.loc.gov/2015040254

RRS1511

Contributors

Monalisa Mullick, MD
Clinical Instructor
Division of Hospital Medicine
Department of Internal Medicine
Washington University School of Medicine
St. Louis, Missouri

Eric Nolley, MD
Pulmonary and Critical Care Fellow
University of Pittsburgh
Pittsburgh, Pennsylvania
Former Internal Medicine Resident
Washington University School of Medicine
St. Louis, Missouri

Jennifer Wilkinson, MD
Assistant Professor
Division of Hospital Medicine
Department of Internal Medicine
Emory University School of Medicine
Atlanta, Georgia

Preface

The academic Hospital Medicine Faculty at Washington University perform well over 1000 bedside procedures per year, the vast majority of which are performed in a teaching capacity. I serve as Director of our Procedure Service, a rotation where interns and residents are supervised performing a variety of invasive procedures. This book is meant to serve as a comprehensive, hands-on guide to performing bedside procedures. We chose procedures commonly performed by most house staff, but especially those in Internal Medicine or Surgery, or those who are enrolled in a preliminary or transitional internship.

I am often asked whether a particular procedure is safe to perform in a patient with an elevated International Normalized Ratio, or thrombocytopenia. We have reviewed the literature regarding "safe" cutoffs for various bedside procedures and, where applicable, summarized these data in the appropriate chapters. Ultimately, the decision to proceed with a procedure will depend on the relative benefits and risks of that procedure in a specific patient, but this book should serve as a good starting point for those decisions.

The use, potential benefits, and technique of ultrasound guidance for certain procedures are also included. Basic interpretation of test results is discussed, but in a more cursory fashion. Ultimately, we hope that readers will find this book very useful as a bedside tool for the preparation, performance, and aftercare of invasive bedside procedures.

James Matthew Freer, MD

Contents

Introduction

UNIVERSAL PROTOCOL AND PRECAUTIONS

- Prior to the procedure, applicable labs, images, and other clinical data should be reviewed.

- Informed consent should be obtained. The indications, contraindications, risks, and benefits of the procedure should be explained to the patient, and the patient should express understanding. If the patient is unable to consent to the procedure, a surrogate may consent on his or her behalf. If no surrogate is available, two physicians may agree that the procedure is urgent or emergent and proceed.

- The site of the procedure should be marked if there is more than one potential location for the procedure. For example, mark the correct side for thoracentesis prior to the procedure.

- With all bedside procedures (excluding intubation), the site of the procedure should be sterilely prepped and draped at a minimum. Sterile gloves should be worn at all times. Additional sterile precautions may be necessary for certain procedures and will be discussed in the appropriate chapter.

- Just prior to the start of the procedure, a time-out should be performed and documented. All participants in the procedure should agree on the identity of the patient, including his or her name and date of birth, as well as the procedure to be performed. All participants should agree on the proper site of the procedure.

1 Central Venous Cannulation

OVERVIEW

This chapter will focus on bedside placement of triple lumen catheters via Seldinger technique. If long-term access is needed, consider other options for central venous catheters.

INDICATIONS

- Emergency resuscitation
- Delivery of caustic medications, such as vasopressors or certain antibiotic or chemotherapeutic agents
- Invasive diagnostics including right heart catheterization and central venous pressure monitoring
- Lack of peripheral access with need for lab monitoring and/or routine IV medications

CONTRAINDICATIONS

- Skin or soft tissue infection at site
- Lack of appropriate target vein secondary to thrombosis or local injury (e.g., clavicular fracture)
- Coagulopathy and thrombocytopenia are relative contraindications. There are no agreed-upon "safe" cutoffs for cannulation at any site.
  - One study reviewed 658 cirrhotic patients with thrombocytopenia and/or coagulopathy. Of note, 146 patients had a platelet count below 50,000 cells/µL:
    - 306 internal jugular (IJ) catheters were placed with a mean international normalized ratio (INR) of 2.7 and a mean platelet count of 83,000. No bleeding complications were noted.
    - 352 subclavian catheters were placed with a mean INR of 2.4 and a mean platelet count of 81,000. One case of hemothorax was reported.[1]

CHOICE OF CANNULATION SITE

The choice between IJ, subclavian, and femoral lines should be based on reducing the risk of procedural complications (pneumothorax [PTX], arterial puncture, and malpositioning) and catheter-related complications (catheter-related bloodstream infections and thrombosis). In general, femoral lines are least preferred due to increased risk of catheter colonization and thrombosis.[2] IJ and subclavian catheters have similar overall rates of catheter-related complications, but the risk of specific complications varies between the two:

- One meta-analysis of over 4000 catheters revealed a 3% risk of arterial puncture with IJ cannulation but only 0.5% with the subclavian approach.[3] Ultrasound (US) guidance can reduce this risk (see below), and IJ may be preferred over subclavian in patients with coagulopathy, as direct pressure can be held if arterial puncture occurs.
- Another meta-analysis showed a two-fold increase in line infection with the IJ vs. subclavian approach.[4] Many other (but not all) studies also show a higher rate of infection with IJ lines, and the Centers for Disease Control and Prevention (CDC) endorses the use of subclavian rather than IJ catheters to minimize infection risk.[5]
- Some references cite a higher rate of PTX with the subclavian approach, with the risk of PTX approaching 3% in some studies.[6] Published rates of PTX complicating IJ cannulation are generally lower, with some sources documenting a risk approaching 0%.[7]

See Table 1-1 for a summary of the advantages and disadvantages of the various insertion sites.

SUPPLIES

The following supplies are required for central venous cannulation:
- Central venous catheter kit (generally triple lumen) including the catheter, guidewire, needles, scalpel, dilator, and lumen caps. Ensure that the catheter is of appropriate length for the proposed insertion site.
- Sterile gloves, gown, cap, mask with eye protection, and full body drape
- 1% lidocaine
- Chlorhexidine skin prep
- Sterile normal saline (NS) flushes
- For US guidance, US machine with vascular probe, sterile probe sleeve, sterile US gel
- Suturing material or other securing device and sterile dressing

CATHETER AND GUIDEWIRE PREPARATION

- Prepare the catheter by removing the temporary lumen caps and replacing with needleless caps, leaving the appropriate lumen uncapped to allow later passage of the guidewire.

TABLE 1-1 **Choice of Cannulation Site**		
Anatomic Approach	**Advantages**	**Disadvantages**
Femoral	• Fastest approach in emergent settings • Simple/superficial anatomic landmarks • High success rate • Does not interfere with resuscitative efforts (i.e., CPR/intubation) • No risk of PTX • US guidance may be used if needed	• Generally advised for short-term access only • Highest rate of infection • Highest rate of thrombosis • Interferes with patient mobility
Internal jugular (IJ)	• Higher success rate for less-experienced operators (especially with US guidance) • Lower risk of PTX as compared to subclavian site • Direct pressure may be applied if bleeding occurs	• Risk of arterial puncture (carotid artery) higher than subclavian site • Landmarks more difficult to identify in obese patients • Higher risk of infection as compared to subclavian site • Uncomfortable for patient • Difficult to maintain dressing adherence
Subclavian	• Can be placed in emergent situations while airway is being established • Lowest infection risk • More comfortable for patient than IJ site • Easier to maintain dressings than IJ site • Easier to identify landmarks in obese patients as compared to IJ site	• Lower success rate than IJ approach for inexperienced operators • US guidance possible but is less commonly used and more difficult to master than for IJ cannulation • Higher rate of PTX as compared to IJ site • Cannot apply direct pressure to the vessel in case of bleeding or arterial puncture

- Flush all lumens with sterile NS to ensure patency.
- Ensure that the guidewire moves freely.

SELDINGER TECHNIQUE FOR CATHETER INSERTION AT ALL SITES

1. Use the introducer to insert the curved end of the guidewire through the needle (Fig. 1-1). Insert the guidewire 10–20 cm, using the

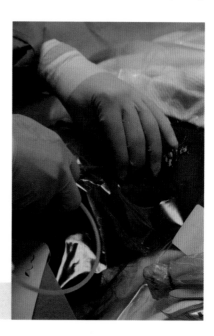

Figure 1-1 Insertion of guidewire through needle.

darker markings to indicate depth. If applicable, US guidance can confirm the presence of the guidewire in the vein (Fig. 1-2). If arterial placement is suspected, follow the steps outlined in the Complications section below.

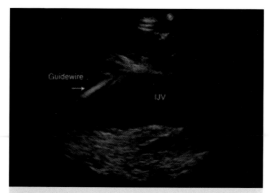

Figure 1-2 Visualization of guidewire in internal jugular vein. IJV, internal jugular vein. (From Barash PG, Cullen BF, Stoelting RK, et al., eds. Clinical Anesthesia. 7th ed. Philadelphia, PA: Wolters Kluwer Health; 2013.)

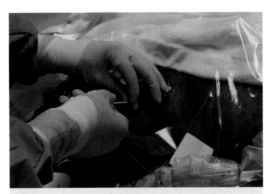

Figure 1-3 Inserting the dilator over the guidewire.

2. **NEVER LET GO OF THE GUIDEWIRE.** Remove the introducer from the free end of the wire and then remove the needle.

3. Nick the skin with the scalpel to allow room for the dilator, taking care to avoid nicking the wire or injuring the vein. Gauze 4 × 4s can be used to minimize the expected increased blood loss from this point until catheter insertion.

4. Taking care to maintain hold of the guidewire, thread the dilator over the wire. Hold the dilator close to the skin, applying gentle forward pressure and rotating to dilate the tract several cm deep (Fig. 1-3).

5. Remove the dilator and thread the catheter over the guidewire. With one hand on the guidewire at all times, back out the guidewire slowly until it exits the distal end of the uncapped catheter lumen (Fig. 1-4). Maintain control of the external end of the guidewire and insert the catheter to the desired depth. Assuming an average-sized patient, depth is as follows:
   - 18 cm for left IJ catheter
   - 17 cm for left subclavian catheter
   - 16 cm for right IJ catheter
   - 15 cm for right subclavian catheter
   - Hub the catheter (generally 20 cm) for femoral insertion

6. While holding the catheter in place, remove the guidewire and confirm it is intact, including the proximal curved end.

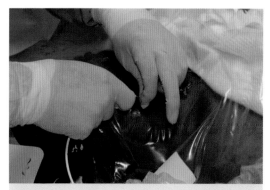

Figure 1-4 Backing the guidewire out of the central venous catheter.

7. Secure the catheter with suture or alternative device (Fig. 1-5).
8. Clean the field with sterile gauze and saline. Dry the area before placing sterile dressing.
9. Obtain a CXR for IJ and subclavian insertion to ensure proper positioning and lack of complications.

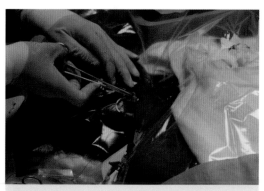

Figure 1-5 Securing the central venous catheter.

INTERNAL JUGULAR APPROACH

PERFORMING THE PROCEDURE

① Obtain informed consent and follow Universal Protocol and Precautions.

② Position the patient supine in bed with chin turned away from the planned access site. Place the bed in Trendelenburg (head-down) 10–15 degrees to improve IJ filling and decrease risk of air embolism.

③ Review landmarks to estimate access point at the apex of the triangle formed by the clavicle, the sternal head of the sternocleidomastoid muscle (SCM), and the clavicular head of the SCM and lateral to the carotid artery. During insertion, direct the needle toward the ipsilateral nipple (Fig. 1-6).

④ Check that all necessary supplies are readily available and functioning properly (see Catheter and Guidewire Preparation above).

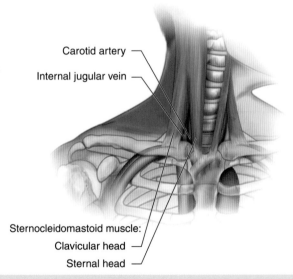

Carotid artery

Internal jugular vein

Sternocleidomastoid muscle:
Clavicular head
Sternal head

Figure 1-6 IJ anatomy and physical examination landmarks. (Modified from Anderson MK. *Foundations of Athletic Training*. 5th ed. Baltimore, MD: Wolters Kluwer; 2012.)

5 US guidance has been shown to reduce the rate of complications compared with landmark guidance alone for IJ catheters.

- A recent Cochrane review showed two-dimensional US reduced the rate of total complications by 71% and arterial puncture by 72%; first attempt success was increased by 57%.[8]

Place the US probe at the estimated insertion site, taking care to localize the left/right indicator on the probe and ensure its position corresponds to the image on the display screen. The vein tends to be larger, collapsible with pressure, and more lateral than the carotid artery, which is generally smaller, with a thicker wall that remains circular and does not collapse with pressure (Fig. 1-7).

6 After marking the insertion site, prep the surrounding field from the clavicle to the earlobe with chlorhexidine. Place the full body drape with adherent dressing surrounding the insertion site, taking care to explain to the patient that room for air flow will be maintained along the contralateral side of the drape. The operator should wear sterile gown, gloves, cap, and mask with eye protection.

7 Perform a "time-out" as detailed in the Introduction.

8 If applicable, prepare the US probe for the sterile field by placing gel on the probe. Cover the probe with a sterile sleeve and secure with

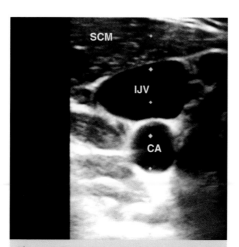

Figure 1-7 US appearance of internal jugular vein and carotid artery. IJV, internal jugular vein; CA, carotid artery.

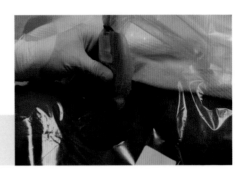

Figure 1-8 Confirming location of IJ with sterile US probe.

rubber band. Apply sterile US gel to the neck and reconfirm proper insertion site (Fig. 1-8).

9 Draw 1% lidocaine into a 5–10-mL syringe using a 21G needle. While confirming position with real-time US guidance, make an SC wheal using a 25G needle. Numb the deeper tissues with the 21G needle, applying gentle suction to the syringe while advancing the needle to ensure that lidocaine is not injected into a vessel.

10 Attach the finder needle to a non-Luer lock syringe. Under US guidance, angle the needle 45 degrees from the skin surface and advance toward the vessel (Fig. 1-9). Remember to apply suction to

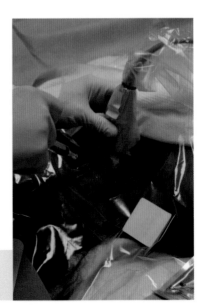

Figure 1-9 Proper angle of insertion for IJ cannulation with US guidance.

the syringe during advancement, and watch for the flash of blood indicating venous access.

- The needle shadow can be visualized entering the vessel using either short-axis/transverse or long axis/longitudinal viewing.[9]

11 Ensure adequate venous flow while drawing back on the syringe, then stabilize the needle with the nondominant hand and remove the syringe. Nonpulsatile darker blood should flow freely. "Flatten" the needle against the skin to allow for easier passage of the guide-wire.

- Observe for signs of arterial puncture (bright red blood, pulsatile flow, or high clinical suspicion). See Complications section below.

See Seldinger Technique for Catheter Insertion at all Sites (p. 4)

SUBCLAVIAN APPROACH

PERFORMING THE PROCEDURE

1 Obtain informed consent and follow Universal Protocol and Precautions.

2 Position the patient supine in bed with chin turned away from the planned access site. Place the bed in Trendelenburg (head-down) 10–15 degrees to improve venous filling and decrease risk of air embolism. A towel roll can be placed under the spine to make the clavicles more prominent, but is generally unnecessary.

3 The subclavian vein courses below the clavicle, superficial and infe-rior to the subclavian artery (Fig. 1-10). Identify the clavicle where

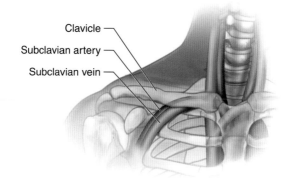

Clavicle
Subclavian artery
Subclavian vein

Figure 1-10 Subclavian vein anatomy. (From Anderson MK. *Foundations of Athletic Training.* 5th ed. Baltimore, MD: Wolters Kluwer; 2012.)

it "bends" more superiorly, generally at a point dividing the medial two-thirds and lateral one-third of the clavicle. The needle will be inserted approximately 2 cm lateral and inferior to this landmark.

4 Check that all necessary supplies are readily available and functioning properly (see Catheter and Guidewire Preparation above).

5 US guidance is also possible at the subclavian site using compressibility and Doppler flow to distinguish between the artery and the vein, although it is not as widely used as for IJ cannulation. This may reduce the risk of arterial puncture and hematoma.[10]

6 After identification of the insertion site, prep a wide field above and below the clavicle with chlorhexidine. Place the full body drape with adherent dressing surrounding the insertion site, taking care to explain to the patient that room for air flow will be maintained along the contralateral side of the drape. The operator should wear sterile gown, gloves, cap, and mask with eye protection.

7 Perform a "time-out" as detailed in the Introduction.

8 Draw 1% lidocaine into a 5–10-mL syringe using a 21G needle. Make an SC wheal at the insertion site with a 25G needle. Numb the deeper tissues with the 21G needle, applying gentle suction to the syringe while advancing the needle to ensure that lidocaine is not injected into a vessel.

9 The angle of insertion of the numbing needle should be fairly superficial and aimed at the "bend" in the clavicle. Reach the clavicle with the numbing needle and then anesthetize the periosteum.

10 Attach the finder needle to a non-Luer lock syringe. Insert the finder needle at the same point as the numbing needle, and advance toward the "bend" in the clavicle. Remember to apply suction to the syringe during advancement.

11 Reach the clavicle with the finder needle, then "walk" the needle down the clavicle in small increments by slowly withdrawing the needle (but not completely out of the skin) and then inserting more posteriorly (i.e., deeply) until the needle slips under the clavicle. The needle should move just beneath the clavicle at a horizontal angle to minimize the risk of PTX.

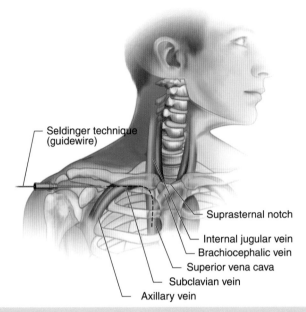

Figure 1-11 Accessing the subclavian vein. (From Anderson MK. *Foundations of Athletic Training.* 5th ed. Baltimore, MD: Wolters Kluwer; 2012.)

Seldinger technique (guidewire)

Suprasternal notch

Internal jugular vein

Brachiocephalic vein

Superior vena cava

Subclavian vein

Axillary vein

12 Once the needle is under the clavicle, redirect the needle, aiming toward the sternal notch (Fig. 1-11). Advance the needle, applying suction to the catheter, until dark, nonpulsatile blood return is obtained. If blood return is not achieved, withdraw the needle but keep it under the clavicle, and redirect either superiorly or inferiorly in small increments until venous blood return is obtained.
  • Observe for signs of arterial puncture (bright red blood, pulsatile flow, or high clinical suspicion). See Complication section below.

13 After blood return, confirm good flow by withdrawing on the syringe. Remove the syringe and rotate the needle 90 degrees inferiorly so that the needle bevel is pointing toward the heart. This will allow for easier guidewire insertion.

See Seldinger Technique for Catheter Insertion at all Sites (p. 4)

FEMORAL APPROACH

PERFORMING THE PROCEDURE

1 Obtain informed consent and follow Universal Protocol and Precautions.

2 Position the patient supine in bed with the leg slightly abducted and externally rotated.

3 Review landmarks to identify the access point. The femoral vein is located medial to the femoral artery and the femoral nerve below the inguinal ligament. Vascular access should occur 1–2 cm below the level of the inguinal ligament and 1–2 cm lateral to the femoral artery pulsation (Fig. 1-12). An assistant or tape can be used to retract any redundant skin or pannus.

4 Check that all necessary supplies are readily available and functioning properly (see Catheter and Guidewire Preparation above).

5 US guidance may be used to lessen the risk of femoral artery puncture. This is uncommon, however, given the often more emergent setting of femoral vein cannulation.

6 After marking the insertion site, prep a wide field around the groin with chlorhexidine. Place the full body drape with adherent dressing surrounding the insertion site. The operator should wear sterile gown, gloves, cap, and mask with eye protection.

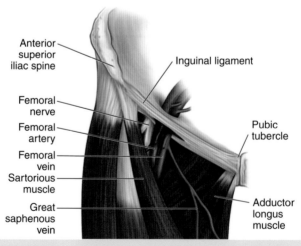

Figure 1-12 Femoral vein anatomy. (From Anderson MK. *Foundations of Athletic Training*. 5th ed. Baltimore, MD: Wolters Kluwer; 2012.)

7 Draw 1% lidocaine into a 5–10-mL syringe using a 21G needle. Make an SC wheal at the insertion site with a 25G needle. Numb the deeper tissues with the 21G needle, applying gentle suction to the syringe while advancing the needle to ensure that lidocaine is not injected into a vessel. The femoral vein can usually be accessed with the 21G needle, but do NOT insert lidocaine into the vessel.

8 Attach the finder needle to a non-Luer lock syringe. Insert the finder needle in the same location and at the same angle as the finder needle. Retract the femoral artery medially with the non-dominant hand to lessen the risk of arterial puncture. Remember to apply suction to the syringe during advancement.

9 Return of dark, nonpulsatile blood should be obtained in the syringe. Confirm adequate blood flow and remove the syringe. "Flatten" the needle against the skin to allow for easier passage of the guidewire.

See Seldinger Technique for Catheter Insertion at all Sites (p. 4)

COMPLICATIONS AND TROUBLESHOOTING

- Arterial puncture can occur at any of the potential cannulation sites. It is critical to recognize arterial puncture before the guidewire is advanced and especially before dilation occurs.
  - Bright red blood is a good indicator of arterial blood unless the patient is hypotensive and/or hypoxic, in which case arterial blood may appear darker.
  - Pulsatile blood is a good indicator of arterial puncture; however, brisk flow can be seen in volume overload states and severe tricuspid regurgitation.
  - If uncertain, connect transduction tubing to the needle, or collect a blood gas to differentiate arterial from venous blood. Venous flow should not be pulsatile or rise to >30 cm hydrostatic pressure (equivalent to 30 mm Hg).
  - For arterial punctures, remove needle and/or guidewire and hold pressure for 10 minutes. US can be used to check for hematomas. If the catheter has been placed, consult surgery for recommendations prior to removal.
- PTX and hemothorax (HTX) are potential complications of IJ and subclavian insertion. If air is aspirated, first check that the syringe is appropriately connected to the needle. If confirmed it is air or the patient is in respiratory distress, abort the procedure and obtain an urgent CXR.

- Difficulty threading the guidewire may indicate vascular thrombus or clot formation in the finder needle. First remove the needle and flush with sterile NS to remove any clots. US may be used to reassess for vascular clot. Do not force the guidewire if it does not pass smoothly.
- If any of the above complications occur during IJ or subclavian line placement, do not attempt placement of central access on the contralateral side at the bedside because of risk of injury to both sides of the chest.

CENTRAL LINE CARE

- Minimizing access to the line and duration of use will help prevent catheter-associated infection. Alcohol preparations to clean hubs and sterile dressing changes should be employed per institutional protocols. Evaluate daily whether the line is still necessary.

REFERENCES

1. Fisher NC, Mutimer DJ. Central venous cannulation in patients with liver disease and coagulopathy—a prospective audit. Intensive Care Med. 1999;25(5):481–5.
2. Ge X, Cavallazzi R, Li C, et al. Central venous access sites for the prevention of venous thrombosis, stenosis, and infection. Cochrane Database Syst Rev. 2012;(3):CD004084.
3. Parienti JJ, du Cheyron D, Timsit JF, et al. Meta-analysis of subclavian insertion and nontunneled central venous catheter-associated infection risk reduction in critically ill adults. Crit Care Med. 2012;40(5):1627–34.
4. Ruesch S, Walder B, Tramér MR. Complications of central venous catheters: internal jugular versus subclavian access—a systematic review. Crit Care Med. 2002;30(2):454–60.
5. O'Grady NP, Alexander M, Burns LA, et al. Guidelines for the prevention of intravascular catheter-related infections, 2011. www.cdc.gov. Accessed 9/18/15.
6. Merrer J, De Jonghe B, Golliot F, et al. Complications of femoral and subclavian venous catheterization in critically ill patients. JAMA. 2001;286(6):700–7.
7. McGee DC, Gould MK. Preventing complications of central venous catheterization. N Engl J Med. 2003;348(12):1123–33.
8. Brass P, Hellmich M, Kolodziej L, et al. Ultrasound guidance versus anatomical landmarks for internal jugular vein catheterization. Cochrane Database Syst Rev. 2015;(1):CD006962.
9. Vogel JA, Haukoos JS, Erickson CL, et al. Is long-axis view superior to short-axis view in ultrasound-guided central venous catheterization? Crit Care Med. 2015;43(4):832–9.
10. Brass P, Hellmich M, Kolodziej L, et al. Ultrasound guidance versus anatomical landmarks for subclavian or femoral vein catheterization [Review]. Cochrane Database Syst Rev. 2015;(1):CD011447.

Radial Arterial Line Placement

INDICATIONS

- Generally accepted indications to perform arterial line placement include:
    - frequent monitoring of pH, P_{O_2}, and P_{CO_2} in patients with respiratory failure
    - hemodynamic monitoring in unstable patients on vasopressors or inotropes
    - patients with inaccurate noninvasive blood pressure monitoring.

CONTRAINDICATIONS

- Absolute contraindications include:
    - traumatic injury proximal to target insertion site
    - infection or burns at the potential insertion site
    - deficient circulation as determined by absent radial pulse or in patients with advanced atherosclerosis
    - Raynaud phenomenon
    - thromboangiitis obliterans.
- Relative contraindications include inadequate collateral flow as determined by Allen test or Doppler ultrasound (US), coagulopathy, or anticoagulation.

SITE SELECTION

- Localization of the radial artery can be performed via palpation or US. Place the patient's hand ventrally on an arm board or bedside table at 30–60 degrees of extension by supporting the dorsal wrist with a support such as a rolled towel or gauze roll. Consider taping the palm and/or wrist to help maintain the wrist in appropriate extension. Optimal palpation of the radial artery is typically between

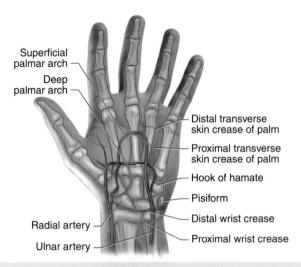

Figure 2-1 Diagram of hand illustrating arterial flow, underlying bony structures, and anatomic structures. (Modified from Anderson MK. *Foundations of Athletic Training*. 5th ed. Baltimore, MD: Wolters Kluwer; 2012.)

the flexor carpi radialis tendon and the radial head 1–2 cm proximal to the wrist (Fig. 2-1).

- If appropriate, assess for collateral flow via the modified Allen test (see Box 2-1).

BOX 2-1

MODIFIED ALLEN TEST

The utility of assessing for collateral flow via the modified Allen test to predict the risk of hand ischemia after catheter insertion is controversial. Perform the modified Allen test by simultaneously occluding both radial and ulnar arteries while having the patient clench and unclench the fist until the palm is blanched, then releasing pressure on the ulnar artery and documenting the time needed for palmar capillary refill to occur. Definitions of abnormal capillary refill time vary from 5 to 15 seconds. Compared with Doppler US, the modified Allen test has moderate diagnostic accuracy and relatively poor specificity for identifying abnormal ulnar blood flow.[1] The Allen test is further limited as critically ill patients are often unable to participate due to sedation or for other reasons. Given the inability of the modified Allen test to predict postcatheterization ischemia, further investigation, that is, with Doppler US or digital plethysmography, should be considered or an alternate site pursued if there is clinical concern.

PERFORMING THE PROCEDURE

1 Obtain informed consent and follow Universal Protocol and Precautions.

2 The arterial line may be placed using either:
- a catheter with a separate guidewire
  or
- an integrated guidewire/catheter device (Fig. 2-2).

3 US guidance for cannulation is often recommended, especially if the radial artery is difficult to palpate or the patient is hypotensive. Meta-analyses of randomized trials comparing palpation vs. real-time US guidance have found that US:
- increases first attempt success
- decreases the number of attempts and time needed for successful cannulation
- decreases hematoma formation in children and adults in both the presurgical and the emergency room settings.[2,3]

4 Either longitudinal or transverse visualization of the radial artery via US can be used depending on operator preference and experience, but one randomized trial found that transverse visualization decreased the number of attempts required for successful cannulation.[4]

5 After identification and marking of the insertion site, prep the area with chlorhexidine and drape the immediate area around the insertion site. The operator should wear sterile gloves, gown, and mask.

6 Perform a "time-out" as detailed in the Introduction.

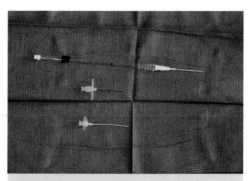

Figure 2-2 Picture of catheter over needle and wire/cook kits.

7 Using the nondominant hand, palpate the radial artery proximal to the insertion site. If using US guidance, use the nondominant hand to hold the US probe and identify the radial artery just proximal to the insertion site.

8 Hold the catheter like a pencil in the dominant hand and insert the catheter into the skin at 45 degrees. If using palpation, advance toward the arterial pulse until blood is observed in the catheter. If using US guidance, advance toward the visualized radial artery until direct cannulation is observed and/or blood is observed in the catheter (Fig. 2-3).

9 If using a catheter over needle device, advance the entire guidewire/needle into the artery with the nondominant hand and then remove the guidewire/needle. If using a device with a wire, insert the wire while holding the needle steady, remove the needle, and then advance the catheter over the wire. Little to no resistance should be met when advancing the wire and or/catheter. If correctly placed, pulsatile flow will be seen, and attaching the pressure transducer will demonstrate an arterial waveform.

10 If the initial attempt is unsuccessful, first reposition the catheter and retry. With successive attempts, once a flash of blood is obtained, attempt to advance the catheter through the artery. Then withdraw the catheter until blood is again seen and advance the guidewire. If arterial vasospasm is suspected, terminate the procedure and pursue an alternate insertion site.

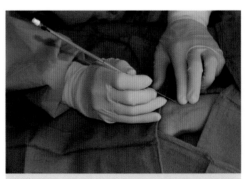

Figure 2-3 Optimal insertion angle with either palpation or US.

⑪ Secure the catheter with suture or other securing device, cleanse the skin and device with antiseptic solution, and cover with an adhesive dressing.

COMPLICATIONS AND POSTPROCEDURE CARE

- Major complications are rare, and most occur at the insertion site. Temporary radial artery occlusion is the most common complication, at approximately 20%, followed by thrombosis.[4] While clinically significant thrombosis is uncommon, occurring in <1%, up to a quarter of patients with arterial lines may develop thrombosis by Doppler US. Thus, arterial lines are routinely flushed with heparin to reduce the risk of thrombosis.

- Other complications include vasospasm, pseudoaneurysm formation, distal ischemia, bleeding, hematoma, iatrogenic blood loss from frequent testing, and local or systemic infection. The risk of infection increases with catheter duration of >4 days.[1,5]

REFERENCES

1. Brzezinski M, Luisetti T, London M. Radial artery cannulation: a comprehensive review of recent anatomic and physiologic investigations. . 2009;109:1763–81.
2. Gao Y, Yan J, Gao F, et al. Effects of ultrasound-guided radial artery catheterization: an updated meta-analysis. 2015;33:50–5.
3. Shiloh A, Savel R, Paulin L, et al. Ultrasound-guided catheterization of the radial artery: a systematic review and meta-analysis of randomized controlled trials. . 2011;139:524–9.
4. Quan Z, Tian M, Chi P, et al. Modified short-axis out-of-plane ultrasound versus conventional long-axis in-plane ultrasound to guide radial artery cannulation: a randomized controlled trial. 2014;119:163–9.
5. O'Horo J, Maki D, Krubb A, et al. Arterial catheters as a source of bloodstream infection: a systemic review and meta-analysis. 2014;42:1334–9.

3 Endotracheal Intubation

OVERVIEW

This chapter is meant to cover the basics of endotracheal intubation. Thus, it is limited in scope as airway management is a subject of significant depth, requiring experience to master. Topics not covered in detail here include the pharmacology of intubation and difficult airway algorithms. Expert consultation from an intensivist or anesthesiologist is necessary if the provider has limited experience or skill.

INDICATIONS

- Acute respiratory failure, hypoxemic and/or hypercarbic
- Cardiopulmonary or respiratory arrest
- To facilitate procedures, for example, esophagogastroduodenoscopy in the setting of acute upper gastrointestinal bleeding
- Upper airway obstruction due to laryngeal edema, mass, or laryngospasm
- Patient inability to maintain/protect airway due to altered mental status from any etiology

CONTRAINDICATIONS

- Penetrating trauma to the upper airway involving the glottis or supraglottic structures, for example, laryngeal fracture, or maxillofacial or oropharyngeal trauma if using an oropharyngeal approach (not all facial trauma is a contraindication to nasal intubation).
- Relative contraindications include severe laryngeal or supralaryngeal edema, pharyngeal mass or foreign body, or a difficult airway exceeding operator experience and/or skill.

PROCEDURE SELECTION

- If endotracheal intubation is contraindicated for any of the above reasons, alternative oxygenation and ventilation strategies including noninvasive or surgical approaches must be considered, depending on the clinical scenario.

- Either direct or indirect laryngoscopy can be performed. Direct laryngoscopy uses a rigid laryngoscope to visualize the vocal cords via direct line of sight. Indirect or video laryngoscopy is performed similarly to direct laryngoscopy, but uses a special laryngoscope (glidoscope, C-mac, etc.) that displays the vocal cords on a video monitor. Studies comparing direct vs. video laryngoscopy indicate that video laryngoscopy may reduce the risk of difficult intubation or esophageal intubation, and increase first attempt success.[1]

- Rapid sequence intubation (RSI) and awake intubation are the two most commonly used approaches. RSI is generally considered the first-line approach in patients with no anticipated difficulties in oxygenation or intubation. Awake intubation is often used in patients anticipated to have a difficult airway. During awake intubation, lighter procedural sedation and analgesics are given, while in RSI larger doses of sedatives and analgesics, in addition to a paralytic agent, are given.

PREPROCEDURAL PREPARATION AND ASSESSMENT

1. Supplies needed (Fig. 3-1)
   a. Bag-valve mask, high-flow oxygen source, suction equipment, laryngoscope handle and blade, endotracheal tube (ETT), stylet, device to confirm ETT placement, and medications. Consider having a laryngeal mask airway (LMA), bougie, and/or other accessory or rescue devices readily available.

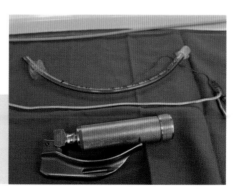

Figure 3-1 Laryngoscope, endotracheal tube, and stylet. (From Chu LF, Fuller A. *A Visual Guide to Anesthesia Procedures.* Philadelphia, PA: Lippincott Williams & Wilkins; 2012.)

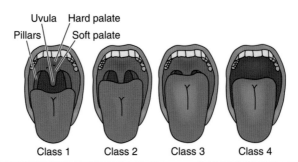

Figure 3-2 Mallampati score used to determine difficulty of airway management. (Modified from Sonnenday CJ, Dimick JB. *Clinical Scenarios in Surgery: Decision Making and Operative Technique*. Philadelphia, PA: Wolters Kluwer; 2012.)

2. Assess for airway difficulty
    a. Factors that may predict a more difficult airway include higher Mallampati class (Fig. 3-2), abnormal dentition, limited neck and/ or jaw mobility, stridor, recent trauma, and history of difficult intubation.
3. Select sedation approach
4. Preoxygenation
    a. Preoxygenation is typically performed via simple nonrebreather (NRB) face mask, high-flow nasal cannula (HFNC), or noninvasive positive pressure ventilation (NIPPV). Healthy subjects will often maintain adequate oxygen saturation for >5 minutes after preoxygenation.[2] Critically ill patients, conversely, are at much greater risk for very rapid desaturation.

PERFORMING THE PROCEDURE

1. Obtain informed consent if possible, and follow Universal Protocol and Precautions.

2. Perform a "time-out" as detailed in the Introduction.

3. Preoxygenate for at least 3 minutes if possible. Note that, depending on the patient and the sedation strategy, preoxygenation may include bag mask ventilation after the patient is sedated.

4. Once sufficiently or maximally preoxygenated, administer chosen sedation approach.

5. Place the patient in the "sniffing" position, which aligns the oral, laryngeal, and pharyngeal axes (Fig. 3-3). To do so, flex the neck approximately 30 degrees, and extend the head at the atlantooccipital joint to 20 degrees.

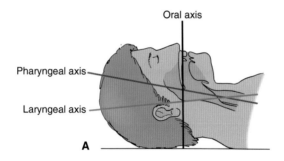

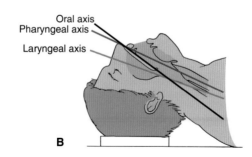

Figure 3-3 Patient pictured in supine anatomical alignment **(A)** and "sniffing position" **(B)**. (Modified from Snell RS. *Clinical Anatomy by Regions.* 8th ed. Baltimore, MD: Wolters Kluwer; 2007.)

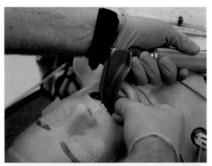

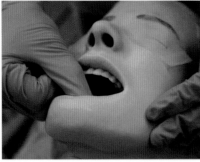

Figure 3-4 Laryngoscope insertion. (From Chu LF, Fuller A. *A Visual Guide to Anesthesia Procedures.* Philadelphia, PA: Lippincott Williams & Wilkins; 2012.)

6 Assuming adequate sedation (and a right-handed operator), use the right thumb and third finger to open the mouth widely via a scissoring motion. With the left hand, insert the laryngoscope blade in the right side of the mouth to the base of the tongue, and gently move the blade to midline, sweeping the tongue from right to left (Fig. 3-4). If done correctly, the laryngoscope handle will be in line with the nasal septum.

7 Advance the blade and expose the vocal cords, elevating the epiglottis by lifting simultaneously upward and forward approximately 45 degrees from the horizontal. Avoid rocking or angulating the laryngoscope handle as doing so often results in dental or oropharyngeal trauma. If the cords are difficult to visualize, consider applying cricoid pressure.

8 After vocal cord visualization (Fig. 3-5), advance the ETT through the right side of the mouth while maintaining view of the cords, whether using direct or indirect laryngoscopy. Advance through the glottis opening until the cuff is no longer visible, and then remove the laryngoscope.

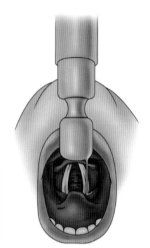

Figure 3-5 Visualization of vocal cords using direct laryngoscopy. (Modified from Hinkle JL, Cheever KH. *Brunner & Suddarth's Textbook of Medical–Surgical Nursing*. 13th ed. Philadelphia, PA: Wolters Kluwer; 2013.)

9 Inflate the cuff with 2–6 mL of air to prevent air leakage during ventilation.

10 Confirm correct placement by assessment for bilateral chest rise, auscultation for bilateral breath sounds, and confirmation by end-tidal CO_2 monitoring.

11 Secure the ETT with adhesive tape.

12 Obtain CXR to confirm appropriate placement.

COMPLICATIONS AND POSTPROCEDURE CARE[3,4]

- Nontraumatic
  - Hypoxemia or hypercarbia due to prolonged intubation attempts. Terminate the attempt once the O_2 saturation is less than 88–90%, given the risk of critical hypoxemia below this level.[2] Intubation attempts should typically last <1 minute.
  - Esophageal intubation or right mainstem bronchus intubation
  - Aspiration of oropharyngeal or gastric contents
  - Bronchospasm or laryngeal spasm
  - Peri-intubation hypertension, arrhythmias, myocardial ischemia or infarction, elevated intracranial pressure or intraocular pressure due to laryngeal stimulation
    - Peri-intubation hypotension due to medications and loss of sympathetic drive

- Traumatic
  - Upper airway trauma (oropharyngeal, laryngeal, or tracheal) including but not limited to vocal cord injury, arytenoid dislocation or subluxation, damage to lips (lacerations), teeth (chipping or avulsion), tongue, esophagus, etc.
  - Temperomandibular joint dislocation
  - Cervical spinal cord injury due to extreme flexion/extension in patients with c-spine pathology

REFERENCES

1. De Jong A, Molinari N, Conseil M, et al. Video laryngoscopy versus direct laryngoscopy for orotracheal intubation in the intensive care unit: a systematic review and meta-analysis. 2014;40:629–39.
2. Weingart S, Levitan R. Preoxygenation and prevention of desaturation during emergency airway management. 2012;59:165–75.
3. Hagberg C, Georgi R, Krier C. Complications of managing the airway. 2005;19:641–59.
4. Pacheco-Lopez P, Berkow L, Hillel A, et al. Complications of airway management. 2014;59:1006–21.

Lumbar Puncture   **4**

INDICATIONS

Lumbar puncture (LP) is indicated urgently for suspected central nervous system (CNS) infection or for suspected subarachnoid hemorrhage (SAH) in a patient with a negative head CT scan. LP may also be needed, though on a more elective basis, to work up a variety of neurological conditions.

CONTRAINDICATIONS AND PREPROCEDURE IMAGING

- Absolute contraindications to LP include infection over the proposed insertion site or suspected lumbar epidural abscess.
- Relative contraindications include thrombocytopenia, coagulopathy, and increased intracranial pressure (ICP). No agreed upon cutoffs for platelet count or international normalized ratio (INR) exist (Table 4-1).
  - One study evaluated over 600 patients with cerebrovascular accident who underwent an LP. Half of the patients were anticoagulated after the LP and half were not. There were no serious bleeding complications in the patients who were not anticoagulated. Conversely, 5 (1.5%) of the anticoagulated patients developed postprocedure paraparesis.[1]
  - Another study evaluated 66 patients with acute leukemia who underwent a total of 195 LPs. The platelet count ranged from 20,000 cells/µL to over 100,000 and included 35 patients with a count between 20,000 and 30,000; no serious bleeding complications were reported.[2]
  - In a small study of cancer patients ($N = 20$) with platelet count <20,000, 2 had postmortem SAH.[3]
  - Aspirin therapy alone is not felt to increase bleeding risk.
  - Case reports of bleeding complications in patients receiving thienopyridine derivatives (e.g., clopidrogel) have been published. However, the magnitude of the bleeding risk in these patients is unknown.

TABLE 4-1 **Bleeding Risk with LP**	
Risk Factor	**Comments**
Platelet count <20,000 cells/µL	• Risks generally outweigh benefits • If LP is deemed necessary, give platelet transfusion prior to procedure • Consider fluoroscopic guidance to lessen bleeding risk
Platelet count 20,000–100,000	• Weigh risks of procedure vs. benefits • Consider platelet transfusion, especially for platelet count <50,000
Coagulopathy or therapeutic anticoagulation	• No generally accepted INR or PTT cutoff • Discontinue IV heparin 2–4 h prior to procedure; wait at least 1–2 h before resuming • Discontinue low-molecular weight heparin 12–24 h prior to procedure • Discontinue warfarin 5–7 d prior to procedure, or give vitamin K and/or fresh frozen plasma to reverse the INR • Discontinue novel oral anticoagulants (NOACs) 12–24 h prior to procedure, depending on the half-life of the drug
Antiplatelet agents	• No increased bleeding risk with aspirin monotherapy • Case reports of bleeding with thienopyridines (e.g., clopidrogel) • Weigh risks and benefits of LP in patients on thienopyridines and discontinue therapy 5–7 d prior to procedure if feasible

PTT, partial thromboplastin time.

- Brain imaging (e.g., CT) is generally not needed prior to LP (see Box 4-1).

BOX 4-1

TO CT OR NOT TO CT?

Two studies evaluated emergency room patients requiring urgent LP. All patients underwent head CT prior to the LP. Only 3–5% of patients had mass effect on brain imaging.[4,5] Predictors of mass effect on CT included altered mental status, focal neurologic findings on physical exam, recent seizure, age >60 (in 1/2 studies), and impaired cellular immunity. Brain imaging prior to LP should be performed in these patients. If mass effect is seen on brain imaging, consult with neurosurgery prior to performing an LP.

PERFORMING THE PROCEDURE

1 Obtain informed consent and follow Universal Protocol and Precautions.

2 Identify appropriate landmarks (Fig. 4-1). A line joining the iliac crests corresponds to the fourth vertebral body. Insertion is generally made at the L3/4 or L4/5 interspace, which is below the spinal cord.

3 Patient positioning is key in successfully obtaining cerebrospinal fluid (CSF). Place the patient in the fetal position, with the neck, back, and legs in flexion to allow widening of the space between the spinous processes. The back should be perpendicular to the bed. The patient may also sit upright, though this precludes measurement of an opening pressure.

4 After marking of the insertion site, prep the area with betadine or chlorhexidine and drape the immediate area around the insertion site. The operator should wear sterile gloves and a mask at a minimum. Concern has been raised over chlorhexidine possibly causing arachnoiditis, although the evidence for this is weak.

5 Perform a "time-out" as detailed in the Introduction, and allow the antiseptic solution to dry.

6 Anesthetize with lidocaine, first by making an SC wheal with a small (25G) needle. Then use a 21G or 22G needle to numb the deeper tissues.

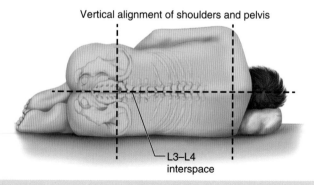

Vertical alignment of shoulders and pelvis

L3–L4 interspace

Figure 4-1 Landmarks for LP. (Modified from Anderson MK. *Foundations of Athletic Training*. 5th ed. Baltimore, MD: Wolters Kluwer; 2012.)

7 Insert a 20G or 22G spinal needle between the spinous processes, usually aimed slightly superiorly toward the umbilicus. Assuming the patient is in the fetal position, the bevel of the needle should be parallel to the bed. Once the superficial tissues are traversed, withdraw the stylet at regular intervals to check for flow of CSF (Fig. 4-2).

8 If bone is encountered, withdraw the needle, but do not entirely remove it from the patient. Adjust the angle of insertion in small increments and again advance the needle. Repeat this process until bone is no longer encountered.

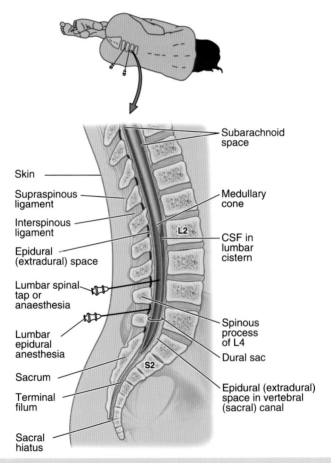

Figure 4-2 Insertion of spinal needle. (Modified from Moore KL, Agur AM, Daley AF. *Essential Clinical Anatomy.* 5th ed. Baltimore, MD: Wolters Kluwer; 2014.)

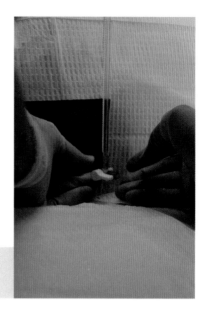

Figure 4-3 Attachment of three-way stopcock to spinal needle and measurement of opening pressure.

9 A "pop" or sensation of decreased pressure may be felt when the needle is inserted past the ligamentum flavum. Once CSF is obtained, connect a three-way stopcock to the spinal needle and measure an opening pressure, if applicable (Fig. 4-3).

10 Collect CSF in tubes. A minimum of 8 mL of CSF is typically collected, although more may be safely removed if specialized tests are required.

11 After CSF collection is complete, insert the stylet back in the spinal needle and remove the needle. Place an adhesive bandage at the insertion site.

COMPLICATIONS AND POSTPROCEDURE CARE

- The most common complications of LP include headache and backache. The following have been shown to reduce the risk of headache:
  - use of a smaller-gauge needle
  - use of an atraumatic rather than cutting needle
  - replacement of the stylet prior to needle removal.

  Bedrest following the procedure has not been shown to reduce headache risk.

- Treatment for post-LP headache includes analgesia and, for refractory cases, an epidural blood patch placed by anesthesia.

- More serious complications of LP include infection (which is rare), spinal hematoma, and cerebral herniation. Risk factors for increased bleeding are outlined in Table 4-1. Prompt diagnosis of a spinal hematoma is key, as emergent spinal decompression is usually required. Cerebral herniation is best prevented by careful patient screening prior to the procedure, as outlined above.

REFERENCES

1. Ruff RL, Dougherty JH. Complications of lumbar puncture followed by anticoagulation. *Stroke*. 1981;12:879–81.
2. Vavricka SR, Walter RB, Irani S, et al. Safety of lumbar puncture for adults with acute leukemia and restrictive prophylactic platelet transfusion. *Ann Hematol*. 2003;82:570–73.
3. Breuer AC, Tyler HR, Marzewski DJ, et al. Radicular vessels are the most probable source of needle-induced blood in lumbar puncture. *Cancer*. 1982;49:2168–72.
4. Hasbun R, Abrahams J, Jekel J, et al. Computed tomography of the head before lumbar puncture in adults with suspected meningitis. *N Engl J Med*. 2001;345:1727–33.
5. Gopal AK, Whitehouse JD, Simel DL, et al. Cranial computed tomography before lumbar puncture: a prospective clinical evaluation. *Arch Intern Med*. 1999;159:2681–85.

Abdominal Paracentesis

INDICATIONS
- Evaluation of new-onset ascites
- Evaluation for suspected spontaneous bacterial peritonitis (SBP)
- Therapeutic removal of ascites in symptomatic patients

CONTRAINDICATIONS
- Absolute contraindications include:
  - bowel obstruction (especially if ultrasound [US] guidance is not used)
  - insufficient ascites
  - skin infection at the proposed insertion site.
- Relative contraindications include thrombocytopenia and coagulopathy. However, paracenteses have been safely performed with an international normalized ratio (INR) as high as 8.7, and a platelet count as low as 19,000.[1] Therefore, blood products are rarely needed prior to the procedure.

PERFORMING THE PROCEDURE

1 Obtain informed consent and follow Universal Protocol and Precautions.

2 Identify and mark ascites at a preferred insertion site, in the far lateral right lower quadrant (RLQ) or left lower quadrant (LLQ) or the midline below the umbilicus (Fig. 5-1; see Box 5-1).

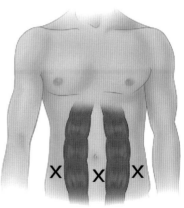

Figure 5-1 Optimal puncture sites for abdominal paracentesis. (Modified from Hinkle JL, Cheever KH. *Brunner & Suddarth's Textbook of Medical-Surgical Nursing*. 13th ed. Philadelphia, PA: Wolters Kluwer; 2013.)

BOX 5-1

ULTRASOUND GUIDANCE

US guidance is generally used to mark the site for paracentesis, but is not absolutely necessary. Use caution to avoid insertion near the liver, spleen, bladder, or inferior hypogastric arteries (Fig. 5-2). US marking was shown in one study to improve success rates, with a 10% absolute increase in successfully obtaining fluid.[2] In the same study, 13/17 patients had successful paracentesis with US marking after an initial failed "blind" attempt. Real-time US guidance is rarely necessary unless the pocket of fluid is extremely small.

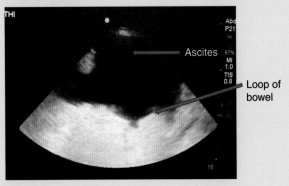

Figure 5-2 US appearance of ascites.

③ After marking of the insertion site, prep the area with chlorhexidine and drape the immediate area around the insertion site. The operator should wear sterile gloves, but full sterile gown, mask, and cap are not necessary.

④ Perform a "time-out" as detailed in the Introduction.

⑤ Draw lidocaine into a 5-mL syringe with a 21G needle. Make an SC wheal with a 25G needle, and numb the deeper tissues with the 21G needle. A "Z-technique" may be used to create a nonlinear pathway between the skin and the peritoneum, minimizing later leakage of ascitic fluid. In all but the most obese patients, ascitic fluid will be obtained using the 21G needle. If the paracentesis is only for diagnostic purposes, fluid may be removed using a different syringe and the procedure is completed.

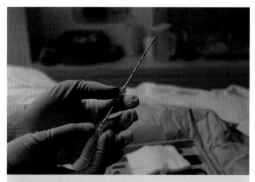

Figure 5-3 Caldwell needle.

6 For therapeutic procedures, the paracentesis needle (generally a Caldwell needle; Fig. 5-3) is then inserted in the same tract, again utilizing a Z-technique. A skin nick using a scalpel may be needed to allow insertion of the paracentesis needle through the skin, although in our experience, this increases the risk of postprocedure ascites leak. Once ascitic fluid is obtained, the needle should be advanced another 1 cm, and the blunt portion of the catheter inserted another several cm over the sharp needle (Fig. 5-4). Free flow of ascitic fluid should be obtained.

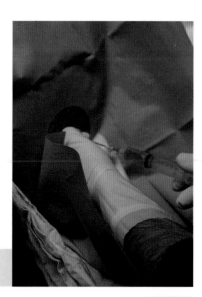

Figure 5-4 Insertion of blunt catheter over Caldwell needle.

7 Fluid for analysis, if desired, should then be obtained (see Box 5-2). Connect the paracentesis needle to appropriate tubing, and remove fluid using either evacuated 1-L glass bottles or suction canisters (Fig. 5-5). If suction canisters are used, connect a three-way stopcock to the catheter to allow flow to be shut off when canisters are changed (Fig. 5-6).

8 If flow terminates or becomes sluggish, bowel or peritoneum may be sucked into the tip of the paracentesis needle. In this case, terminate suction, withdraw the needle in short increments, and resume suction. The patient may also be turned to the side of insertion to facilitate flow, or pressure may be applied to the opposite side of the abdomen to push fluid toward the paracentesis needle.

9 After the desired amount of fluid has been removed, withdraw the paracentesis needle in a swift fashion and apply a Band-Aid or pressure dressing to the site.

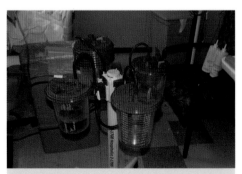

Figure 5-5 Suction canisters used to collect ascites.

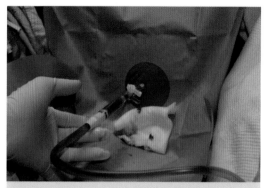

Figure 5-6 Three-way stopcock and suction tubing.

COMPLICATIONS AND POSTPROCEDURE CARE

- Complications, including infection, are rare. Bowel perforation occurs very rarely and can usually be managed conservatively. Bleeding is also uncommon, ranging from 0 to 1% in several case series.[1,3,4]

- The use of albumin following large-volume paracentesis to prevent postparacentesis circulatory dysfunction and possibly acute kidney injury remains controversial, but is endorsed by the American Association for the Study of Liver Diseases. Albumin is given at a dose of 6–8 g/L removed; albumin infusion is generally felt to be unnecessary if less than 5 L was drained.

REFERENCES

1. Grabau CM, Crago SF, Hoff LK, et al. Performance standards for therapeutic abdominal paracentesis. *Hepatology*. 2004;40(2):484.
2. Nazeer SR, Dewbre H, Miller AH. Ultrasound-assisted paracentesis performed by emergency physicians vs the traditional technique: a prospective, randomized study. *Am J Emerg Med*. 2005;23:363–7.
3. Pache I, Bilodeau M. Severe haemorrhage following abdominal paracentesis for ascites in patients with liver disease. *Aliment Pharmacol Ther*. 2005;21:525.
4. De Gottardi A, Thévenot T, Spahr L, et al. Risk of complications after abdominal paracentesis in cirrhotic patients: a prospective study. *Clin Gastroenterol Hepatol*. 2009;7:906.

6 Thoracentesis

INDICATIONS

- Indications for diagnostic thoracentesis include sampling of a new pleural effusion, especially if infection is suspected (see Box 6-1). Suspected transudates can be observed, but thoracentesis should be considered if the effusion does not improve as expected with diuresis.

- A therapeutic thoracentesis should be considered in patients with shortness of breath attributable to the pleural effusion.

CONTRAINDICATIONS

- Use extra caution when performing a thoracentesis in patients with coagulopathy, thrombocytopenia, or uremic platelet dysfunction.
  - Bleeding risk is not increased in patients with an international normalized ratio (INR) as high as 2.0, or a platelet count as low as 50,000/μL.

BOX 6-1

FLUID ANALYSIS

Pleural effusions are classified as transudates or exudates. Although newer classification schemes have been proposed, Light's criteria are still most generally used to distinguish the two (Table 6-1). Light's criteria are extremely sensitive for the diagnosis of a transudate but less specific. Diuresis of a transudative effusion may lead to a falsely elevated pleural protein level, which is called a *pseudoexudate*. If a transudative effusion is strongly suspected clinically, the serum to pleural fluid albumin gradient may be calculated. A gradient of >1.2 g/dL is very specific for a transudative effusion.

TABLE 6-1 Light's Criteria

Pleural Fluid LD Classification	Pleural/Serum Protein Ratio	Pleural/Serum LD Ratio	Pleural Fluid (ULN)
Transudate	<0.5	<0.6	<2/3
Exudate	≥0.5	≥0.6	≥2/3

An effusion is exudative if any of Light's criteria is met.
LD, lactate dehydrogenase; ULN, upper limit of normal reference range for serum LD.

- Preprocedure blood products have not been shown to decrease bleeding risk.
- One study reviewed 1009 ultrasound (US)-guided thoracenteses in patients with coagulopathy and/or thrombocytopenia. 248 of these patients had a platelet count <50,000/μL, and the mean INR was 1.9. Approximately 30% of patients were given blood products prior to thoracentesis. Only four cases of bleeding were reported, all in patients who received prophylactic blood products.[1]

PERFORMING THE PROCEDURE

1 Obtain informed consent and follow Universal Protocol and Precautions.

2 Position the patient upright if possible, leaning over a bedside tray. If the patient is unable to sit upright, position the patient in the lateral decubitus position. Physical exam should confirm the presence of a pleural effusion, with decreased breath sounds and dullness to percussion of the appropriate lower lung field.

3 Review pertinent imaging studies, including CXR and CT.

4 Ultrasound guidance has become standard of care when performing a thoracentesis, either utilizing real-time imaging or by placing a mark at the appropriate site (Fig. 6-1).

- One small but widely cited study showed a decrease in the rate of pneumothorax (PTX) from a baseline of 8.6→1.1% after physicians underwent US training.[2]
- A much larger retrospective review revealed a 3.1% risk of PTX in "blind" thoracentesis vs. 2.3% with US guidance.[3]

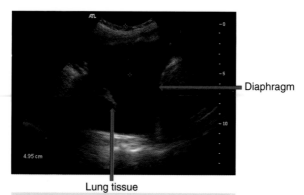

Figure 6-1 US appearance of pleural effusion.

- The use of US guidance likely increases thoracentesis success rates. In one small study, 88% of patients had a successful US-guided procedure after an initial dry "blind" attempt.[4]

5 After marking of the insertion site, prep the area with chlorhexidine and drape the immediate area around the insertion site. The operator should wear sterile gloves at a minimum.

6 Perform a "time-out" as detailed in the Introduction.

7 Draw lidocaine into a 5–10 mL syringe using a 21G needle. Make an SC wheal using a 25G needle, and numb the deeper tissues with the 21G needle (usually 3.5–4 cm in length). Insert the needle perpendicular to and above the rib to minimize the risk of bleeding.

8 Pleural fluid can often be obtained with the 21G needle, in which case lidocaine can be injected into the pleural space. If the thoracentesis is only for diagnostic purposes, fluid may be removed using a different syringe and the procedure is completed.

9 For therapeutic procedures, make a skin nick with a scalpel at the insertion site.

10 Insert the thoracentesis catheter, again making sure that it is superior and perpendicular to the rib. Once fluid is obtained in the syringe, insert the catheter another 1 cm, then advance the blunt and flexible catheter another several cm over the needle (Fig. 6-2). Advance the catheter such that all of the openings on the distal catheter are within the pleural space.

11 Remove the needle and connect the catheter to appropriate tubing. Fluid is usually withdrawn in a syringe and then injected through a two-way valve into a collection bag (Fig. 6-3).

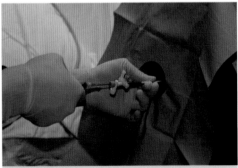

Figure 6-2 Insertion of blunt catheter over needle.

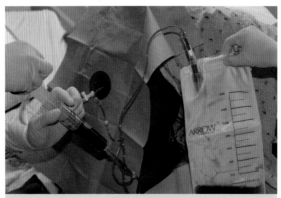

Figure 6-3 Pleural fluid collection system.

12 If flow becomes sluggish, withdraw the catheter in small increments to see if flow improves. Terminate the procedure if flow does not improve.

13 Some coughing during the procedure is expected as the lung and pleura reexpand. Reasons to terminate the procedure include:
- aspiration of blood when the fluid was not initially bloody
- aspiration of air
- severe pain or shortness of breath
- intractable cough.

14 Removal of 1.5 L or sometimes more pleural fluid is felt to be safe, although the risk of reexpansion pulmonary edema and especially PTX may increase with greater fluid removal.[5]

15 When fluid removal is completed, close the catheter system to the patient, and ask the patient to Valsalva by exhaling or humming as the catheter is removed.

COMPLICATIONS AND POSTPROCEDURE CARE

- The risk of PTX varies widely in published studies, but seems to be diminished in the era of US guidance. Bleeding occurs in <1% of patients.

- In the absence of signs or symptoms of PTX, a postprocedure CXR is not needed. In one study, only 4/488 asymptomatic patients had a PTX on chest imaging, and only one of these required a chest tube.[6]

REFERENCES

1. Hibbert RM, Atwell TD, Lekah A, et al. Safety of ultrasound-guided thoracentesis in patients with abnormal preprocedural coagulation parameters. 2013;144:456–63.
2. Duncan DR, Morgenthaler TI, Ryu JH, et al. Reducing iatrogenic risk in thoracentesis: establishing best practice via experiential training in a zero-risk environment. 2009;135:1315–20.
3. Mercaldi CJ, Lanes SF. Ultrasound guidance decreased complications and improves the cost of care among patients undergoing thoracentesis and paracentesis. . 2013;143:532–38.
4. Kopman DF. Ultrasound-guided thoracentesis. 2006;129:1709–14.
5. Josephson T, Nordenskjold CA, Larsson J, et al. Amount drained at ultrasound-guided thoracentesis and risk of pneumothorax. 2009;50:42.
6. Alemán C, Alegre J, Armadans L, et al. The value of chest roentgenography in the diagnosis of pneumothorax after thoracentesis. 1999;109:340–3.

Knee Arthrocentesis 7

INDICATIONS

Diagnostic:

- Assessment of suspected septic arthritis
- Initial confirmation of gouty arthritis
- Evaluation of joint effusion of unclear etiology

Therapeutic:

- Relief of pain by aspirating effusion or blood
- Injection of medications (e.g., corticosteroids, antibiotics, or anesthetics)
- Drainage of septic effusion

CONTRAINDICATIONS

- Cellulitis at the site of needle entry
- Known or suspected bacteremia (relative)
- Prosthetic joints (relative contraindication due to increased risk of iatrogenic infection)[1]
- There are no contraindications to sampling and drainage of a suspected septic joint.
- Knee aspiration appears safe in patients receiving therapeutic anticoagulation and/or antiplatelet agents. Caution should be taken in patients with supratherapeutic anticoagulation as the upper limit of a "safe" Internationalized Normalized Ratio (INR) is unknown.[2–4]

SUPPLIES

- Skin cleansing agent (betadine or chlorhexidine)
- Numbing agent (Ethyl chloride spray or 1% lidocaine)
- Small needle (i.e., 25G) for numbing
- Larger needle (i.e., 18G–21G 1.5-inch needle)
- One 5 mL syringe and one or two 30 mL syringes
- Sterile drape
- Gloves
- Hemostat
- Sterile gauze

- Device to mark insertion site, such as a pen or the sterile end of a needle cap
- Collection tubes for cell count, culture, and crystal analysis, as appropriate
- Sterile steroid preparation (if applicable)

CHOICE OF ASPIRATION/INJECTION SITE

The choice of insertion site depends on several factors, including the patient's anatomy and the ease of palpating a joint effusion at each site, the patient's ability to flex or extend the knee, and operator experience and preference. See Figures 7-1 through 7-3 for knee anatomy.

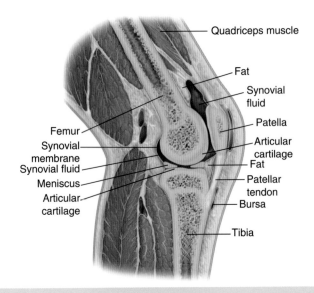

Figure 7-1 Anatomy of the knee. (Modified from Creason C. *Stedman's Medical Terminology*. Baltimore, MD: Wolters Kluwer; 2010.)

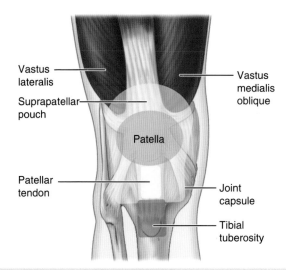

Figure 7-2 Anterior view of knee and surrounding structures. (Modified from Anderson MK. *Foundations of Athletic Training*. 5th ed. Baltimore, MD: Wolters Kluwer; 2012.)

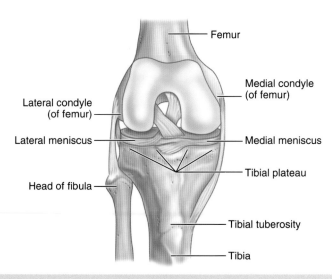

Figure 7-3 Bony anatomy of the knee. (Modified from Anderson MK. *Foundations of Athletic Training*. 5th ed. Baltimore, MD: Wolters Kluwer; 2012.)

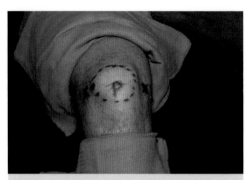

Figure 7-4 Lateral or medial midpatellar insertion approach. Points of insertion are marked with an "X."

1. Lateral or medial midpatellar or patellofemoral approach (Fig. 7-4):
   - Traditionally the most commonly used approach
   - Performed with knee in extension
   - Pull the patella opposite the side of insertion.
   - Insert needle 1 cm lateral to the midpoint of the patella, aimed under the patella at the contralateral patellar midpoint.[5]

2. Superolateral or superomedial (i.e., suprapatellar) approach (Fig. 7-5):
   - Useful if a large effusion in the suprapatellar bursa is suspected (communicates with the joint space in the vast majority of patients).

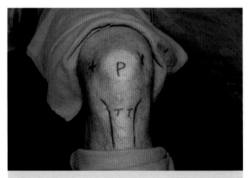

Figure 7-5 Superolateral or superomedial (i.e., suprapatellar) insertion approach. Points of insertion are marked with an "X."

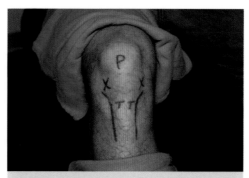

Figure 7-6 Inferolateral or inferomedial (i.e., infrapatellar) approach. Points of insertion are marked with an "X."

- Performed with patient supine and knee in 15–20 degrees of flexion. Often, a towel roll is placed under the knee to facilitate flexion.
  - i. For superolateral approach, insert needle 1 cm superior and 1 cm lateral to the superolateral aspect of the patella.[6]
  - ii. For superomedial approach, insert needle 1 cm superior and 1 cm medial to the superomedial aspect of the patella.
- Advance needle under the patella toward the intercondylar notch of the femur.

3. Inferolateral or inferomedial (i.e., infrapatellar) approach (Fig. 7-6):
   - Useful if the knee cannot be extended, or if only a small amount of fluid is suspected.[5]
   - Performed with knee flexed
   - Insert needle laterally or medially to the patellar tendon.
   - Advance needle superiorly toward the femoral notch.

PERFORMING THE PROCEDURE

1 Palpate the knee to choose an appropriate insertion site as outlined above.

2 Prep the skin with either povidone-iodine or chlorhexidine and place a drape around the insertion site. Shaving the site prior to the procedure is not needed.[3]

3 Perform a "Time-out" as detailed in the Introduction.

4 Anesthetize the skin with either ethyl chloride spray, a topical anesthetic, or 1% lidocaine. Ethyl chloride spray is marked nonsterile, although no increased risk of infection has been associated with its use.[7]

5 If using lidocaine for anesthesia, make a wheal at the insertion site with a 25G needle attached to a 5 mL syringe. Advance the needle into the skin in the planned trajectory of arthrocentesis. Apply suction to the syringe before injecting lidocaine to ensure that it is not injected into a vessel.

6 Attach an 18G or 21G needle to a 30 mL syringe. Insert the needle in the same trajectory as the numbing needle, withdrawing on the syringe during advancement. Flow of synovial fluid should ensue. We often begin with a 21G needle, although if the fluid is viscous with sluggish flow, a larger-bore needle will be necessary. Avoid contact with bony surfaces during insertion, as it can lead to increased pain and damage to chondral cartilage.[5]

7 Remove as much fluid as possible. If needed, use a hemostat to grip the needle and change syringes. "Milking" the effusion by pushing inferiorly in the suprapatellar area may aid in fluid removal.

8 If applicable, after aspiration is complete change the syringe and inject steroid into the joint space.

9 Remove the needle, cleanse the skin with an alcohol wipe, and apply a bandage.

COMPLICATIONS AND TROUBLESHOOTING

Approach to the "dry tap":

- Causes[8]:
  1. Lack of synovial fluid
  2. Extra-articular needle placement during aspiration
  3. Deep effusion with insufficient needle length
  4. High-viscosity fluid or debris encountered by needle tip
- Troubleshooting after a dry tap:
  1. Attempt arthrocentesis at a different insertion site. The operator may use the nondominant hand, or an assistant, to compress the fluid toward the needle from the opposite side of the joint.
  2. Utilize ultrasound (US) guidance to confirm presence and depth of the effusion (see Box 7-1).
  3. Consider aspiration of the joint under fluoroscopic guidance.

Complications:

- Bleeding is rare in the absence of severe thrombocytopenia or coagulopathy.
- Infection is also rare, occurring in less than 1/3000 procedures.[12]

BOX 7-1

ULTRASOUND GUIDANCE

Literature advocating the use of US for knee arthrocentesis is growing. The benefits of US guidance include[5,9,10]:

- Increased aspiration success
- Greater amount of synovial fluid removed with more complete joint decompression[10]
- Decreased postprocedural pain
- Increased efficacy of medications injected into the joint space
- Less damage to articular structures

US may be used for marking of a large effusion to aid in proper needle insertion, or for direct visualization and aspiration of a smaller effusion.

- Indirect approach:
  1. Visualize the effusion via US. The midpoint of the US image corresponds to the middle of the US probe.
  2. Make note of the depth of the effusion and the angle of the US probe against the skin.
  3. Mark the skin at the midpoint of the US probe.
  4. Insert the needle for joint aspiration and/or injection at the skin mark in the same angle as the US probe, keeping in mind the depth required to reach effusion.[11]
- Direct approach:
  1. Apply sterile gel to the skin and to the US probe. Cover the probe with a sterile sleeve.
  2. Hold the US probe to the skin with the nondominant hand, and hold the 18G or 21G needle with the dominant hand.
  3. Identify the effusion, noting its depth, and insert the needle at the midpoint of the US probe, at the same angle as that of the probe.
  4. The needle will appear as a bright white line and can be visualized entering the effusion.[11]

- Increased pain following the procedure may suggest puncture of articular structures.
- Although not an avoidable complication, large effusions may accumulate rapidly following arthrocentesis.[1]
- Joint instability rarely ensues after repeated corticosteroid injections. Thus, injections should be given no more frequently than every 6–8 wks, and no more than three times per year.[1]

See Box 7-2 for information regarding fluid analysis.

BOX 7-2

JOINT FLUID ANALYSIS

Joint fluid may be sent for Gram stain and culture, crystal analysis, white blood cell (WBC) count, and other specialized studies, depending on the clinical scenario. Consult with the laboratory prior to aspiration to confirm that fluid is placed in the appropriate tubes.

- Crystal analysis can confirm the presence of urate (gout) crystals or calcium pyrophosphate dihydrate (pseudogout) crystals.
- The joint fluid WBC is useful in determining the likelihood of bacterial infection. A cell count <25,000/µL decreases the risk of bacterial infection with a likelihood ratio (LR) of 0.32. Conversely, the risk of bacterial infection rises with increasing cell count, with a LR of 2.9, 7.7, and 28 for cell counts >25,000, 50,000, and 100,000/µL, respectively.[13]
- A higher percentage of neutrophils, particularly >90%, in the joint fluid makes bacterial infection more likely.
- The Gram stain reveals organisms in 50–70% of cases of nongonococcal septic arthritis.[14]

REFERENCES

1. Zuber TJ. Knee joint aspiration and injection. *Am Fam Physician*. 2002;66(8):1497–501.
2. Thomsen TW, Shen S, Shaffer RW, et al. Arthrocentesis of the knee. *N Engl J Med*. 2006;354:19.
3. Roberts WN Jr. Joint aspiration or injection in adults: technique and indications. In: Furst DE, ed. *UpToDate*. Waltham, MA: UpToDate; 2015.
4. Ahmed I, Gertner E. Safety of arthrocentesis and joint injection in patients receiving anticoagulation at therapeutic levels. *Am J Med*. 2012;125(3):265–9.
5. Douglas RJ. Aspiration and injection of the knee joint: approach portal. *Knee Surg Relat Res*. 2014;26(1):1–6.
6. Maricar N, Parkes MJ, O'Neill TW. Where and how to inject the knee—a systemic review. *Semin Arthritis Rheum*. 2013;43(2):195–203.
7. Polishchuk D, Gehrmann R, Tan V. Skin sterility after application of ethyl chloride spray. *J Bone Joint Surg Am*. 2012;94(2):118–20.
8. Roberts WN, Hayes CW. Joint aspiration: the dry tap. In: Furst DE, ed. *UpToDate*. Waltham, MA: UpToDate; 2014.
9. Berkoff DJ, Miller LE, Block JE. Clinical utility of ultrasound guidance for intra-articular knee injections: a review. *Clin Interv Aging*. 2012;7:89–95
10. Sibbitt WL Jr, Kettwich LG, Band PA, et al. Does ultrasound guidance improve the outcomes of arthrocentesis and corticosteroid injection of the knee? *Scand J Rheumatol*. 2012;41(1):66–72.
11. Bruyn GAW. Musculoskeletal ultrasonography: guided injection and aspiration of joints and related structures. In: Shmerling RH, ed. *UpToDate*. Waltham, MA: UpToDate; 2014.

12. Geirsson AJ, Statkevicius S, Víkingsson A. Septic arthritis in Iceland 1990–2002: increasing incidence due to iatrogenic infections. *Ann Rheum Dis.* 2008;67(5):638.
13. Margaretten ME, Kohlwes J, Moore D, et al. Does this adult patient have septic arthritis? *JAMA.* 2007;297(13):1478–88.
14. Schmerling RH. Synovial fluid analysis: a critical reappraisal. *Rheum Dis Clin North Am.* 1994;20(2):503.